THE VOICE OF YOUR BODY

The Inner Symphony, Harmonizing Health Through Body Awareness; Unlocking The Music Of Your Body

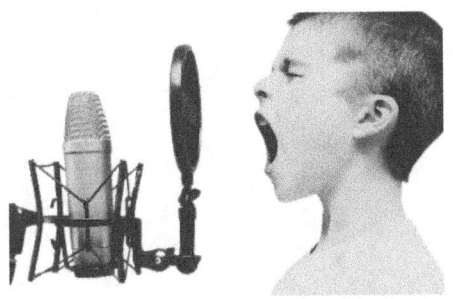

Damaris Roberts

THE VOICE OF YOUR BODY

The Inner Symphony, Harmonizing
Health Through Body Awareness;
Unlocking The Music Of Your Body

Damaris Roberts

Copyright [2024] [Damaris Roberts]

All rights reserved.

The information presented in this book is for general informational purposes only and is not intended to be a substitute for professional medical advice, diagnosis, or treatment. The author is not a medical professional, and the content of this book should not be used as a replacement for consultation with a qualified healthcare provider.

This book is protected by copyright law. No part of this book may be reproduced, stored in a retrieval system, or transmitted in any form or by any means, electronic, mechanical,recording,photocopying,

or otherwise, without the prior written permission of the author.

Damaris Roberts

2024

TABLE OF CONTENTS

6–DISCLAIMER
7–THE PURPOSE OF THIS BOOK
10–INTRODUCTION
12–UNDERSTANDING THE HARMONY OF YOUR BODY
16–YOUR BODY'S DAILY SYMPHONY
18–THE LANGUAGE OF YOUR BODY
21–CHAPTER ONE
21–The Orchestra Members
    The body systems
21–THE HEART- The tireless drummer
25–CHAPTER TWO
25–THE LUNGS: The flutes of life
28–CHAPTER THREE
28–THE DIGESTIVE SYSTEM
31–CHAPTER FOUR
31–THE MUSCULAR SYSTEM
35–CHAPTER FIVE
35–THE SKELETAL SYSTEM
38–CHAPTER SIX
38–THE NERVOUS SYSTEM
41CHAPTER SEVEN
41–THE ENDOCRINE SYSTEM
44–CHAPTER EIGHT
44–THE LIVER
47–CHAPTER NINE
47–THE KIDNEYS

50–CHAPTER TEN
50–THE SKIN
55–CHAPTER ELEVEN
55–THE IMMUNE SYSTEM
60–A HARMONIOUS BODY
61–CHAPTER TWELVE
61–THE BODY'S LANGUAGE
83–LISTENING AND RESPONDING
85–CHAPTER THIRTEEN
85–NUTRITION, HYDRATION AND EXERCISE
93–CHAPTER FOURTEEN
93–MENTAL HEALTH
94–MIND-BODY CONNECTION
97–CONCLUSION
101–A LIFELONG PROCESS
102–REFLECTIONS
104–ABOUT THE AUTHOR
105–YOUR FEEDBACK
106–OTHER BOOKS BY DAMARIS ROBERTS

DISCLAIMER

The information provided in "The Voice of Your Body" is for educational and informational purposes only. While the author has made every effort to ensure accuracy, this book is not written by a medical professional and should not be used as a substitute for professional medical advice, diagnosis, or treatment. Always consult with a healthcare provider before making any changes to your health regimen or if you have any concerns about a medical condition. The author and publisher disclaim any liability for any adverse effects resulting directly or indirectly from the use of the information contained in this book.

THE PURPOSE OF THIS BOOK

"The Voice Of Your Body" is crafted to take readers on an extraordinary journey through the interrelated symphony that exists in the human body. As the author, my intention is to showcase the beauty, complexity, and harmony of each bodily system, likening them to an orchestra where every member plays a vital role in the grand performance of life. This book is not just a scientific exploration; it is a celebration of the body's remarkable capabilities and the fascinating ways in which it maintains health and balance.

What the readers will gain:

After perusing through this book, the readers are expected to:

1. Appreciate more, the harmony of the body's systems by:

a- Understanding how each system, from the heart and lungs to the immune and endocrine systems, works in perfect harmony to sustain life.

b- Recognize the interdependence of these systems, much like the sections of an orchestra, creating a balanced and cohesive whole.

2. Identify the signs and symptoms of these elements by:

a- Learning to listen to their body's whispers, cries, and shouts, recognizing early warning signs of potential health issues.

b- Gaining insight into the significance of

various symptoms and the appropriate actions to take in response.

3. Explore the factors affecting your health by:

a- Discovering how nutrition, hydration, exercise, rest, and mental health impact the body's performance.

b- Understanding the obstacles that can hinder the body's systems and learn strategies to overcome them.

4. Implement preventive measures and maintenance practices by:

a - Embracing a lifestyle that supports ongoing health and wellness, incorporating daily habits that promote balance and vitality.

b- Incorporating the importance of preventive measures, such as regular check-ups, vaccinations, and mindful living.

5. Connect their mind and body by:

a - Realizing the powerful connection between mental and physical health, exploring practices like mindfulness and meditation to maintain overall well-being.

b- Appreciating the role of stress management and emotional health in sustaining the body's harmony.

6. Celebrate the journey of health after all by:

a- Feeling empowered to take charge of
their health, armed with knowledge and practical tips to support their body's unique needs.
b- Celebrating their own body's symphony,
understanding and respecting the signals it sends and the care it requires.

This book is directed to educate, inspire, and empower readers, transforming their understanding of the body from a mere collection of parts to a masterful orchestra, each system playing its unique part in the magnificent performance of life.

Let's kick off to a better health, to a newer version of ourselves!

INTRODUCTION

Welcome to Your Body's Orchestra

Dear reader, as we take off this journey together, I want you to visualize your body as a grand orchestra, each system and organ an instrument playing in harmony to create the music of life. Just like in an orchestra, where every instrument must be in tune and play its part, every part of your body must work together seamlessly. This book is your backstage pass to understanding the incredible performance happening within you every day. It is of great importance that you take note of every information that would guide you on a recovery mission of your overall health after this adventure. You must keep the music of your body beating to the desired tune. Every research that I have made has been to generate updated ideas on the part we have to play as humans to keep the rhythm of our lives going.

Let us picture our body in this way:

Your heart is the tireless drummer, keeping a steady beat day and night. while the lungs are the flutes, filling you with the breath of life. The digestive system is the bass section, breaking down food to provide energy with the mumbling and tumbling accompanying it as it works to break down food particles. Muscles are the string section, promoting movement and strength. And your bones are the percussion, providing structure and support. The nervous system is the conductor, ensuring every part knows when to play its part. And let's not forget the immune system, the choir that defends against invaders, and the skin, your protective barrier. Sounds funny! Right? But that's what goes on everyday in our body system.

UNDERSTANDING THE HARMONY OF YOUR BODY:

Every second, your body performs countless functions that keep you alive and healthy. These functions are so well-coordinated that we often take them for granted. Yet, each system has a voice, a way of communicating when things are going well or when there is trouble. Understanding these voices and learning to listen to them is crucial for maintaining good health. Let us introduce these performers one by one:

The Heart: The tireless drummer

The heart beats about 100,000 times a day, pumping blood throughout your body. This blood delivers oxygen and nutrients to cells and removes waste products. When the heart is healthy, it keeps a steady, strong rhythm. However, if it is overworked or faces issues like high blood pressure or cholesterol buildup, it may signal trouble through symptoms like chest pain or shortness of breath.

The Lungs: The flutes of life

Your lungs take in oxygen and expel carbon dioxide, a crucial process for survival. Every breath you take is part of this life-sustaining melody. If your lungs face challenges like infections, allergies, or chronic conditions like asthma, they may 'speak' through coughing, wheezing, or difficulty in breathing.

The Digestive System: The bass section
Digesting food is a complex symphony involving several organs, including the stomach, intestines, liver, and pancreas. These organs work together to break down food, absorb nutrients, and expel waste. When something disrupts this process, you might experience symptoms like stomach pain, bloating, or changes in bowel habits.

The Muscular System: The string section
Muscles are responsible for movement and maintaining posture. They work by contracting and relaxing, much like the strings of a violin. Regular exercise keeps muscles strong and flexible. However, injuries, overuse, or conditions like arthritis can cause muscles to become stiff or weak, leading to pain and limited movement.

The Skeletal System: The percussion zone
Your bones provide structure and protect vital organs. They also produce blood cells and store minerals. Keeping your bones healthy involves adequate calcium intake, regular exercise, and avoiding activities that increase the risk of fractures. Conditions like osteoporosis can weaken bones, making them more susceptible to fractures.

The Nervous System: The conductor
The nervous system controls and coordinates all bodily functions. It comprises the brain, spinal cord, and nerves, acting as the conductor of your body's orchestra. It sends and receives signals, ensuring that everything runs smoothly. When the nervous system faces challenges like injury, stress, or neurodegenerative diseases, it can lead to symptoms like pain, numbness, or impaired movement.

The Endocrine System: The harmonic chords
The endocrine system produces hormones that regulate many bodily functions, including metabolism, growth, and mood. These hormones act as the harmonic chords that keep your body in balance. If the endocrine system is disrupted, it can cause hormonal imbalances leading to issues like weight gain, fatigue, or mood swings.

The Immune System: The body's defense choir
The immune system protects your body from harmful invaders like bacteria, viruses, and other pathogens. It acts as a choir, singing in unison to defend against infections. A strong immune system is crucial for staying healthy. However, if it is weakened or overactive, it can lead to frequent infections or autoimmune diseases.

The Skin: The protective barrier
Your skin is the first line of defense against external threats. It acts as a barrier, protecting your internal

organs from harmful substances and pathogens. Keeping your skin healthy involves regular cleansing, moisturizing, and protecting it from excessive sun exposure. Conditions like eczema or infections can compromise your skin's integrity, leading to discomfort or other health issues.

YOUR BODY'S DAILY SYMPHONY

Every day, your body performs a symphony of functions that keep you alive and well. Here are some fascinating facts about what happens in your body on a daily basis:

1. Cellular activity: Your body produces millions of new cells every second. These cells replace old or damaged ones, ensuring that your tissues and organs function properly.

2. Digestive process: On average, your digestive system processes about 2.5 liters of food and drink each day. It breaks down nutrients, absorbs them into your bloodstream, and expels waste products.

3. Blood circulation: Your heart pumps approximately 7,500 liters of blood through your body daily. This blood travels through a network of blood vessels that, if laid end-to-end, would stretch around and around multiple times.

4. Respiratory function: You take about 20,000 breaths each day, inhaling oxygen and exhaling carbon dioxide. This process is essential for providing energy to your cells.

5. Nervous system activity: Your brain processes billions of bits of information every second. It controls everything from your thoughts and emotions to your movements and bodily functions.

6. Muscle movement: Even when you are at rest, your muscles are constantly working. They help maintain your posture, support your organs, and enable you to move when needed.

THE LANGUAGE OF YOUR BODY

Your body has a unique way of communicating its needs and issues. It 'speaks' through various signs and symptoms, letting you know when something is wrong or when it needs attention. Learning to interpret these signals is crucial for maintaining good health. Some of these signs are:

1. Pain: Pain is your body's way of signaling that something is wrong. It can be caused by injury, inflammation, or underlying health conditions. Paying attention to pain and seeking medical advice when necessary is important.

2. Fatigue: Feeling excessively tired or fatigued can indicate various issues, such as lack of sleep, poor nutrition, or underlying health conditions like anemia or thyroid problems.

3. Digestive issues: Symptoms like bloating, constipation, or diarrhea can signal problems with your digestive system. Identifying and addressing these issues can improve your overall well-being.

4. Skin changes: Changes in your skin, such as rashes, discoloration, or dryness, can indicate underlying health issues. Keeping your skin healthy involves proper care and attention to any changes.

5. Mood swings: Hormonal imbalances, stress, or mental health issues can cause mood swings. Paying attention to your mental and emotional health is as important as taking care of your physical health.

THE VOICE OF YOUR BODY

THE ROLE OF LIFESTYLE CHOICES

Your lifestyle choices play a significant role in how well your body functions. Here are some key areas to focus on:

1. Nutrition: Eating a balanced diet rich in fruits, vegetables, whole grains, and lean proteins provides the nutrients your body needs to function optimally. Avoiding processed foods, excessive sugar, and unhealthy fats can prevent many health issues.

2. Hydration: Staying hydrated is crucial for maintaining bodily functions. Drinking enough water helps regulate body temperature, aids digestion, and keeps your skin healthy.

3. Exercise: Regular physical activity strengthens your muscles, improves cardiovascular health, and boosts your immune system. Aim for at least 150 minutes of moderate exercise per week.

4. Sleep: Getting enough restful sleep is essential for overall health. Aim for 7-9 hours of sleep per night to allow your body to repair and rejuvenate.

5. Stress management: Chronic stress can negatively impact your health. Practicing stress-reducing techniques like meditation, deep breathing, and spending time in nature can help maintain a healthy mind and body.

In conclusion, understanding the intricate symphony of functions within your body is key to maintaining good health. By listening to your body's signals, making healthy lifestyle choices, and seeking medical advice when necessary, you can ensure that your body's orchestra continues to play a harmonious tune. In this book, you will learn more about each system, how they communicate, what can hinder their functions, and how to keep them in optimal condition. Welcome to "The Voice of Your Body"! Let's embark on this journey to a better health together. This is just the beginning!

CHAPTER ONE

The Orchestra Members - The body systems

We have displayed the framework of this exciting manuscript in the introductory part, now we are in to uncover all about these acting members of the orchestra of our body. Together, we are going to study about how they work and how we can manage them properly too. Their functions to us depend also on the care we give them. Let us embark on this journey with curiosity because we must get the best at the end. Firstly, we are diving into one of the major organs of the body - the heart.

THE HEART- The tireless drummer

Imagine the heart as the tireless drummer of your body's orchestra, setting the pace for everything you do. This incredible organ beats around 100,000 times a day, tirelessly pumping blood through a vast network of blood vessels. It is a muscular marvel about the size of your fist, nestled snugly in your chest.

Each heartbeat sends a surge of blood, rich with oxygen and nutrients, to every part of your body. The heart has four chambers: two atria on top and two ventricles below. Blood flows into the atria from the body and lungs, then it's pumped out from the ventricles to the lungs and the rest of the body. The right side of the heart handles deoxygenated blood, sending it to the lungs for oxygenation, while the left side pumps oxygen-rich blood to the body.

WHAT SLOWS DOWN THE DRUMMER?

Despite its strength, the heart can face challenges that slow its rhythm or make its beat uneven. Here are some common issues:

a-High blood pressure (hypertension): When blood pressure is consistently too high, it forces the heart to work harder, which can lead to damage over time. It is like making the drummer play faster and harder than it is meant to. If you are a dancer, you know also how difficult it seems to make steps when your favorite music turns into a fast tantrum. You will always sweat it out. Picture the overworked heart that way. If you danced and got exhausted and left the hall to catch some breath, what about the stressed heart- our body's kind drummer? Let's keep the rthym moving! We will get this and give our best to our hearts.

b-Cholesterol buildup: Cholesterol can build up in the arteries, forming plaques that narrow the passageways for blood. This can lead to conditions like atherosclerosis, reducing the efficiency of blood flow and making the heart work harder.

c- Heart attack: If an artery supplying the heart with blood becomes blocked, part of the heart muscle can become damaged or die. This is a heart attack, and it is akin to the drummer missing a crucial beat in the orchestra.

d-Arrhythmias: These are irregular heartbeats that disrupt the heart's rhythm. They can make the heart beat too fast, too slow, or erratically, causing symptoms like palpitations, dizziness, or fatigue.

HOW TO KEEP THE BEAT STRONG:
Maintaining a healthy heart involves lifestyle choices and sometimes medical intervention. Here are some ways to keep your heart drumming along:

a-Healthy diet: Eating a diet low in saturated fats, trans fats, cholesterol, and sodium can help keep your arteries clear and blood pressure in check. Include plenty of fruits, vegetables, whole grains, and lean proteins in your diets.

b-Regular exercise: Physical activity strengthens the heart muscle, improves blood circulation, and helps maintain a healthy weight. Aim for at least 150 minutes of moderate exercise per week.

c-Avoid smoking: Smoking damages blood vessels, raises blood pressure, and contributes to plaque buildup in the arteries. Quitting smoking can significantly improve heart health.

d-Stress management: Chronic stress can negatively impact heart health. Practice relaxation techniques like deep breathing, meditation, or yoga to keep stress levels in check.

e-Regular check-ups: Routine medical check-ups can help monitor blood pressure, cholesterol levels, and overall heart health, allowing for early detection and management of potential issues. Always visit your professional health care provider when you feel any sign of ill health.

CHAPTER TWO

THE LUNGS: The flutes of life

Next in our orchestra, we have the lungs, the delicate flutes of life, playing a crucial role in your body's melody. With every breath you take, your lungs fill with air, extract oxygen and expel carbon dioxide, keeping the air fresh for your body's needs. This vital gas exchange keeps your cells energized and your body functioning.

Your lungs are a pair of spongy, air-filled organs located in your chest. They work in harmony with the diaphragm, a dome-shaped muscle at the bottom of the ribcage. When you inhale, the diaphragm contracts and flattens, creating a vacuum that pulls air into the lungs. When you exhale, the diaphragm relaxes, pushing air out of the lungs.

WHAT CHOKES THIS MELODY?

The lungs are delicate instruments, and several factors can disrupt their function, choking the melody they play. Here's some:

a-Respiratory infections: Conditions like pneumonia, bronchitis, and the flu can cause inflammation and infection in the lungs, making it difficult to breathe and reducing oxygen intake.

b-Asthma: This chronic condition causes the airways to become inflamed and narrow, leading to wheezing, shortness of breath, and coughing. It is like a flute player struggling to blow air through a partially blocked instrument.

c-Chronic Obstructive Pulmonary Disease (COPD): This includes emphysema and chronic bronchitis, often caused by long-term exposure to irritating gas or particulate matter, most commonly from cigarette smoke. It damages the airways and alveoli (tiny air sacs in the lungs), making it hard to breathe.

d-Allergies: Allergens like pollen, dust, and pet dander can trigger respiratory symptoms in sensitive individuals, leading to congestion, sneezing, and difficulty breathing.

HOW TO KEEP THE FLUTES CLEAR AND STRONG:

To ensure your lungs stay healthy and your breathing remains smooth, consider these strategies:

a-Avoid smoking: Smoking is the leading cause of lung disease. Quitting smoking can dramatically improve lung health and reduce the risk of chronic obstructive pulmonary disease, lung cancer, and other respiratory conditions.

b-Stay active: Regular physical activity helps improve lung capacity and efficiency. Even activities like walking, swimming, and yoga can benefit lung function.

c-Breathe clean air: Minimize exposure to pollutants, allergens, and secondhand smoke. Use air purifiers at home if necessary and avoid areas with high levels of air pollution.

d-Practice deep breathing: Techniques like diaphragmatic breathing and pursed-lip breathing can help increase lung capacity and improve oxygen exchange.

e-Get vaccinated: Vaccines can protect against respiratory infections like the flu and pneumonia, reducing the risk of serious lung infections or complications.

CHAPTER THREE

THE DIGESTIVE SYSTEM

The bass section breaking down the symphony of food

The digestive system is similar to the bass section in our body's orchestra. It lays down the foundational rhythms of our health by processing the food we eat, extracting vital nutrients and energy, much like how the bass provides depth and support to the music.

The journey of digestion begins in the mouth, where food is chewed and mixed with saliva. It then travels down the esophagus to the stomach, where stomach acids break it down further. From the stomach, the semi-digested food moves into the small intestine, where most nutrient absorption occurs. The large intestine absorbs water and forms waste products, which are then expelled from the body. Can't you see so great a machinery our body inhabits. This book offers insight to us to appreciate these organs more than we do in order to enhance their performance.

WHAT CAUSES THE BASS TO FALTER?

Several factors can disrupt the smooth operation of the digestive system, causing discomfort and health issues.Let's pick some examples:

a-Poor diet: Diets high in processed foods, unhealthy fats, and sugars can lead to digestive problems like constipation, indigestion, and bloating. It is like feeding the bass section out-of-tune notes, causing a discordant sound.

b-Lack of fiber: Fiber is essential for healthy digestion. It adds bulk to stool and aids in its passage through the digestive tract. A low-fiber diet can lead to constipation and other digestive issues.

c-Dehydration: Water is crucial for digestion, helping to dissolve nutrients and soften stool. Not drinking enough water can slow down the digestive process and lead to constipation.

d-Stress: Chronic stress can affect digestion, leading to symptoms like stomach pain, nausea, and changes in appetite. Stress hormones can interfere with the normal contractions of the digestive tract.

e-Infections and diseases: Conditions like irritable bowel syndrome (IBS), Crohn's disease, and infections like gastroenteritis can cause significant digestive distress.

HOW TO TUNE BACK YOUR DIGESTIVE SYSTEM:

Keeping your digestive system in optimal condition requires a combination of healthy eating habits, hydration, and lifestyle choices. They are as follows:

1-Balanced diet: Add a variety of fruits, vegetables, whole grains, lean proteins, and healthy fats in your diet. Avoid excessive consumption of processed foods, sugars, and unhealthy fats.

2-High-fiber foods: Incorporate fiber-rich foods like beans, lentils, whole grains, fruits, and vegetables to promote healthy digestion and prevent constipation.

3-Stay hydrated: Drink plenty of water throughout the day to aid digestion and maintain regular bowel movements.

4-Mindful eating: Eat slowly and chew your food thoroughly. Avoid eating large meals late at night and try to have a consistent eating schedule.

5-Stress management: Practice relaxation techniques like yoga, meditation, or deep breathing exercises to reduce stress and its impact on your digestive system.

6-Probiotics: Probiotics are beneficial bacteria that support gut health. Include probiotic-rich foods like yogurt, kefir, sauerkraut, and other fermented foods in your diet.

CHAPTER FOUR

THE MUSCULAR SYSTEM

The String Section

The muscles in your body are the string section of your orchestra, responsible for the powerful movements and graceful motions you perform daily. From lifting heavy objects to fine motor skills like writing, your muscles play a crucial role. Have you ever seen a guitarist playing with loose strings?

The melody is always affected.

Muscles are an integral part of the human body that helps in mobility and general activities.

Your body has three types of muscles: skeletal, smooth, and cardiac. Skeletal muscles are attached to bones and are responsible for voluntary movements. Smooth muscles are found in the walls of internal organs and control involuntary movements, such as digestion. Cardiac muscles are found only in the heart and are responsible for pumping blood. What a perfect fitting, and we need not to unbalance this setting.

WHAT CAUSES THE STRINGS TO BREAK?

Muscles can face several challenges that weaken or damage them, disrupting their function. Here are examples:

a-Injuries: Strains, sprains, and tears can occur from overexertion, improper use, or accidents. These injuries can cause pain, swelling and limited mobility, much like a broken string on a guitar.

b-Overuse: Repetitive motions or overuse of certain muscle groups can lead to conditions like tendinitis or muscle fatigue, making the muscles sore and less efficient.

c-Lack of use: Inactivity or a sedentary lifestyle can cause muscles to weaken and shrink, a condition known as atrophy. It is like leaving a guitar unplayed, leading to a loss of its fine tuning.

d-Nutritional deficiencies: Muscles require adequate nutrients, especially protein, to repair and grow. A poor diet lacking essential nutrients can hinder muscle health and recovery.

d-Chronic conditions: Diseases such as muscular dystrophy, arthritis, and other chronic conditions can affect muscle function and strength, leading to persistent pain and disability.

HOW TO TUNE YOUR MUSCLES UP

Maintaining strong and flexible muscles requires a combination of regular exercise, proper nutrition, and healthy habits:

1-Regular exercise: Engage in a balanced exercise routine that includes strength training, cardiovascular activities, and flexibility exercises. Aim for at least 150 minutes of moderate exercise per week.

b-Proper form: Use correct techniques when lifting weights or performing exercises to avoid injuries. Consider working with a fitness trainer to ensure proper form.

c-Warm-up and Cool-down: Always warm up before exercising to prepare your muscles and cool down afterward to prevent stiffness and soreness.

d-Balanced diet: Consume a diet rich in proteins, healthy fats, and carbohydrates to provide the necessary fuel and building blocks for muscle repair and growth.

e-Stay hydrated: Drink plenty of water before, during, and after exercise to keep muscles hydrated and functioning optimally.

f-Rest and Recovery: Allow time for muscles to rest and recover between workouts. Overworking muscles can lead to injuries and hinder progress.

Dear reader, will you agree with me that our major challenge in our body maintenance is not the knowledge of what to do but the failure to do it? This book displays the totality of all we need to do to keep the symphony of our system kicking right and we can not help but grab these tips and tricks for our benefits. Sickness and diseases are inevitable when they land on our body for a reason beyond our control but if we become health conscious, adapt to some positive lifestyle uncovered here, our body will sing and dance a balanced rhythm more than before.

CHAPTER FIVE

THE SKELETAL SYSTEM

The percussion section

Your skeletal system is the percussion section of your body's orchestra, providing structure, support, and protection. This system comprises 206 bones, and it is the framework that supports your body, allowing you to stand, move, and perform daily activities. It also plays crucial roles in producing blood cells and storing essential minerals like calcium and phosphorus.

Bones are dynamic tissues that continuously remodel themselves. They consist of a hard outer layer (cortical bone) and a spongy inner layer (trabecular bone), which houses bone marrow.

WHAT DAMPENS THE BEAT?

The skeletal system can face several challenges that weaken or damage bones, affecting their ability to support and protect.

Below are some factors that triggers the malfunctioning:

a-Osteoporosis: This condition weakens bones, making them fragile and more prone to fractures. It is like a drum with a cracked surface, unable to produce a strong, steady beat.

b-Fractures: These are breakages in the bone caused by trauma or accidents which can disrupt the integrity and function of the skeletal system.

c-Arthritis: This inflammation of the joints can cause pain, stiffness, and reduced mobility, much like dampened drum beats in the percussion section.

c-Nutritional deficiencies: Lack of essential nutrients like calcium and vitamin D can weaken bones and hinder their ability to repair and grow.

d-Lack of physical activity: Inactivity can lead to bone loss and decreased bone density, much like an unused drum losing its tension and resonance.

KEEPING THE BEAT STRONG

Maintaining strong and healthy bones requires a combination of proper nutrition, regular exercise, and healthy lifestyle choices:

a-Balanced diet: Consume foods rich in calcium and vitamin D, such as dairy products, leafy greens, and fortified foods. These nutrients are essential for bone health and strength.

b-Regular exercise: Engage in weight-bearing exercises like walking, jogging, and strength training to stimulate bone growth and maintain bone density.

c-Avoid smoking and excessive alcohol: Smoking and excessive alcohol consumption can weaken bones and increase the risk of fractures.

d-Safety measures: Take precautions to prevent falls and injuries, especially as you age. Ensure your home is safe and free of tripping hazards.

e-Regular check-ups: Regular bone density tests and medical check-ups can help monitor bone health and detect issues early.

CHAPTER SIX

THE NERVOUS SYSTEM

The Conductor

The nervous system is the conductor of your body's orchestra, the command center, coordinating and controlling every function and response. It consists of the brain, spinal cord, and a vast network of nerves that transmit signals throughout the body. The brain, the master conductor, processes information and sends commands, while the spinal cord and nerves act as communication pathways. What a co- ordination! Imagine a beautiful choir singing in different parts,the alto,the soprano, the tenor, all making melody to the audience. It would be a wonderful exhibition. That's what goes on when the central nervous system is working in unity, beating in tune uninterrupted.

WHAT CAUSES THE CONDUCTOR TO FALTER?

The nervous system can face several challenges that disrupt its function and communication, leading to a breakdown in the body's coordination. These obstructions can be in form of:

a-Injuries: Trauma to the brain or spinal cord can cause significant damage, leading to loss of function or paralysis. It is like a conductor being unable to direct the orchestra, thereby causing chaos.

b-Neurodegenerative diseases: Conditions like Alzheimer's, Parkinson's, and multiple sclerosis gradually damage the nervous system, leading to symptoms like memory loss, tremors, and impaired movement.

c-Infections: Infections like meningitis or encephalitis can inflame the brain and spinal cord, disrupting their function and causing severe symptoms.

d-Chronic conditions: Conditions like diabetes can damage nerves over time, leading to neuropathy and loss of sensation.

e-Mental health issues: Stress, anxiety, and depression can affect the brain's function, leading to symptoms like fatigue, mood swings, and impaired concentration.

HOW TO KEEP THE CONDUCTOR SHARP

Maintaining a healthy nervous system involves a combination of mental and physical health practices, nutrition, and lifestyle choices. Examples are:

a-Mental stimulation: Keep your brain active with activities like reading, puzzles, and learning new skills. Mental stimulation helps maintain cognitive function.

b-Physical exercise: Regular exercise improves blood flow to the brain, supports nerve health, and helps manage stress.

c-Healthy diet: Consume a balanced diet rich in omega-3 fatty acids, antioxidants, and vitamins to support brain health. Include foods like fish, nuts, berries, and leafy greens in your diets.

d-Sleep: Adequate sleep is essential for brain health and function. Aim for 7-9 hours of quality sleep each night.

e-Stress management: Practice relaxation techniques like meditation, deep breathing, and yoga to reduce stress and its impact on the nervous system.

f-Safety measures: Protect your head and spine with appropriate safety gear during activities like sports and biking to prevent injuries.

CHAPTER SEVEN

THE ENDOCRINE SYSTEM

The Harmonic chords

The endocrine system is the harmonic chords of your body's orchestra, producing hormones that regulate numerous bodily functions. These hormones act as chemical messengers, controlling processes like metabolism, growth, mood, and reproductive health.

The endocrine system comprises glands such as the thyroid, pituitary, adrenal glands, and pancreas. These glands release hormones directly into the bloodstream, which then travel to target organs and tissues. Imagine a group of teens setting the stage in order for a music presentation. There is no need for a breakage, they pass information one to the other.

WHAT THROWS OFF THE HARMONY?

Several factors can disrupt the balance of the endocrine system, affecting hormone production and function. Let us consider these;

a-Hormonal imbalances: Conditions like hypothyroidism, hyperthyroidism, and diabetes result from imbalances in hormone levels, causing symptoms like fatigue, weight changes, and mood swings.

b-Chronic stress: Prolonged stress can lead to overproduction of stress hormones like cortisol, disrupting the balance of other hormones and affecting overall health.

c-Nutritional deficiencies: Lack of essential nutrients can hinder hormone production and function, much like missing notes in a chord.

d-Age-related changes: Hormone levels naturally decline with age, affecting metabolism, mood, and overall health.

e-Environmental toxins: Exposure to certain chemicals and toxins can interfere with hormone production and disrupt the endocrine system.

MAINTAINING HARMONIC BALANCE

Keeping the endocrine system in harmony involves a combination of healthy eating, stress management, and regular medical care:

a-Balanced diet: This is a factor that prevails in every aspect of the function of the body system in order to keep the orchestra in tune. Consume a diet rich in whole foods, including plenty of fruits, vegetables, whole grains, and lean proteins. Avoid processed foods and excessive sugar intake.

b-Regular exercise: Physical activity helps regulate hormone levels, improve metabolism, and reduce stress.

c-Stress management: Practice relaxation techniques and prioritize self-care to manage stress and support hormonal balance.

d-Adequate sleep: Ensure you get enough quality sleep to support hormone production and overall health.

e-Regular check-ups: Routine medical check-ups and blood tests can help monitor hormone levels and detect imbalances early.

CHAPTER EIGHT

THE LIVER

The detox maestro

The liver is the detox maestro of your body's orchestra, the body's detoxifier, responsible for filtering toxins, metabolizing nutrients, and producing essential proteins. This vital organ plays a key role in digestion, detoxification, and overall metabolism.

The liver processes everything you ingest, food, drinks, medication, breaking down harmful substances and converting nutrients into forms the body can use. It also produces bile, which helps digest fats.

WHAT OVERLOADS THIS DETOX MAESTRO?
Several factors can impair liver function, leading to health issues. They are:

a-Excessive alcohol consumption: Drinking too much alcohol can cause liver inflammation and damage, leading to conditions like fatty liver disease, hepatitis, and cirrhosis.

b-Poor diet: A diet high in fats, sugars, and processed foods can contribute to fatty liver disease and other liver conditions.

c-Infections: Viral infections like hepatitis B and C can cause chronic liver inflammation and damage.

d-Medications and toxins: Overuse of certain medications, exposure to industrial chemicals, and ingestion of toxic substances can harm the liver.

e-Obesity: Excess body weight can lead to non-alcoholic fatty liver disease, where fat accumulates in the liver.

HOW TO SUPPORT THE DETOX MAESTRO

To maintain a healthy liver, adopt these liver-friendly habits:

a-Moderate alcohol consumption: Limit alcohol intake to prevent liver damage. If you have liver disease, avoid alcohol altogether.

b-Healthy diet: Eat a balanced diet rich in fruits, vegetables, whole grains, and lean proteins. Avoid high-fat, high-sugar, and processed foods.

c-Stay hydrated: Drink plenty of water to support liver function and overall detoxification.

d-Exercise regularly: Regular physical activity helps maintain a healthy weight and supports liver health.

e-Avoid toxins: Minimize exposure to environmental toxins and follow medication guidelines to prevent liver damage.

f-Regular check-ups: Regular medical check-ups and liver function tests can help monitor liver health and detect issues early.

CHAPTER NINE

THE KIDNEYS

The filters of life

The kidneys are the purifying filters of your body's orchestra, responsible for removing waste products and excess fluids from the blood. These bean-shaped organs play a crucial role in maintaining fluid balance, regulating blood pressure, and supporting overall health.

Each kidney contains millions of tiny filtering units called nephrons, which filter blood, remove waste, and produce urine. The kidneys also balance electrolytes and produce hormones that regulate blood pressure and red blood cell production.

WHAT CLOGS THE FILTERS?

Several factors can impair kidney function, leading to health issues. Let's look at some examples:

a-Dehydration: Inadequate fluid intake can reduce kidney function and increase the risk of kidney stones and urinary tract infections.

b-High blood pressure: Hypertension can damage blood vessels in the kidneys, impairing their ability to filter blood effectively.

c-Diabetes: High blood sugar levels can damage the kidneys over time, leading to diabetic nephropathy.

d-Infections: Recurrent urinary tract infections and kidney infections can damage kidney tissue and reduce function.

e-Medications and toxins: Overuse of certain medications and exposure to toxins can harm the kidneys.

HOW TO MAINTAIN THE FILTERS

To maintain healthy kidneys and optimal filtration function, adopt these habits:

a-Stay hydrated: Drink plenty of water to support kidney function and prevent dehydration.

b-Healthy diet: Eat a balanced diet low in sodium, processed foods, and sugars. Include foods rich in potassium and other essential nutrients.

c-Monitor blood pressure: Keep blood pressure under control through diet, exercise, and medication if needed.

d-Manage diabetes: If you have diabetes, manage blood sugar levels to prevent kidney damage.

e-Avoid overuse of medications: Follow medication guidelines and avoid overusing painkillers and other drugs that can harm the kidneys.

f-Regular check-ups: Regular medical check-ups and kidney function tests can help monitor kidney health and detect issues early.

CHAPTER TEN

THE SKIN

The protective barrier

The skin is the body's largest organ in terms of space, acting as the protective barrier in our orchestra of bodily functions. It serves as the first line of defense against external threats, regulates temperature, and allows us to feel sensations. This remarkable organ is composed of three main layers: the epidermis, dermis, and subcutaneous tissue, each playing a crucial role in maintaining overall health. Let's break down these layers:

THE LAYERS OF PROTECTION

1. Epidermis: The outermost layer, the epidermis, is composed primarily of keratinocytes, which produce keratin, a protein that provides strength and waterproofing. This layer also contains melanocytes, which produce melanin, the pigment responsible for skin color and protection against UV radiation.

2. Dermis: The middle layer, the dermis, houses blood vessels, nerves, hair follicles, and sweat glands. It provides structural support and elasticity, thanks to the collagen and elastin fibers found here.

3. Subcutaneous Tissue: The innermost layer, also known as the hypodermis, consists of fat and connective tissue that insulates the body and cushions internal organs.

WHAT THREATENS THIS BARRIER?

Several factors can impair the skin's function and health, leading to various skin conditions:

a- UV Radiation: Excessive exposure to ultraviolet (UV) rays from the sun can damage skin cells, leading to sunburn, premature aging, and an increased risk of skin cancer.

b-Dehydration: Inadequate water intake can lead to dry, flaky skin and reduced elasticity, making the skin more susceptible to damage.

c-Pollution: Environmental pollutants can clog pores, leading to acne and other skin irritations. Long-term exposure can also accelerate aging and contribute to skin diseases.

d-Poor nutrition: A diet lacking essential nutrients can affect skin health, causing conditions like acne, eczema, and psoriasis.

e-Stress: Chronic stress can exacerbate skin conditions, leading to flare-ups of acne, eczema, and psoriasis.

f-Infections: Bacterial, viral, and fungal infections can cause a range of skin issues, from mild irritations to severe diseases.

NURTURING THE PROTECTIVE BARRIER

To maintain healthy skin and ensure it functions effectively as a protective barrier, adopt these skincare habits:

a-Sun protection: Use broad-spectrum sunscreen with at least SPF 30 daily, even on cloudy days. Wear protective clothing and seek shade during peak sun hours.

b-Hydration: Drink plenty of water to keep the skin hydrated and maintain its elasticity. Hydrated skin is better able to heal and defend itself against external threats.

c-Healthy diet: Eat a balanced diet rich in vitamins, minerals, and antioxidants. Foods high in vitamin C, vitamin E, and omega-3 fatty acids are particularly beneficial for skin health.

d-Gentle skincare routine: Cleanse the skin with gentle, non-irritating products. Avoid harsh soaps and chemicals that can strip the skin of its natural oils.

e-Moisturize: Use a moisturizer suitable for your skin type to maintain hydration and protect the skin's barrier function.

f-Manage stress: Practice stress-reducing techniques such as yoga, meditation, and regular exercise to help maintain healthy skin.

g-Avoid smoking: Smoking accelerates skin aging and increases the risk of skin diseases. Avoid smoking and exposure to secondhand smoke.

h-Regular check-ups: Monitor your skin for any changes or abnormalities. Regular dermatological check-ups can help detect issues early and prevent serious conditions.

LISTENING TO THE SKIN'S VOICE

The skin communicates with us through various signs and symptoms, indicating when something is amiss. Let's hear them:

a-Dryness: Dry, flaky skin may indicate dehydration or a need for more moisturizing products. It can also be a sign of underlying health conditions like hypothyroidism or diabetes.

b-Redness and irritation: Red, inflamed skin can be a response to allergens, irritants, or infections. Identifying and avoiding triggers is crucial.

c-Breakouts: Acne and other breakouts can be caused by hormonal changes, stress, poor diet, or inadequate skincare routines.

d-Changes in moles or spots: Any changes in size, shape, or color of moles or skin spots should be examined by a dermatologist, as they could indicate skin cancer.

e-Itching: Persistent itching can be a sign of allergies, infections, or underlying conditions such as liver disease or kidney problems.

By paying attention to these signals and taking proactive steps to care for the skin, we can ensure this vital organ continues to protect us and contribute to our overall well-being.

CHAPTER ELEVEN

THE IMMUNE SYSTEM

The Body's defense choir singing away the invaders

Envisage your body as a grand concert hall, and within its walls, there exists a choir unlike any other. This choir, the immune system, is dedicated to defending the body from countless invaders. Every note they sing, every harmony they create, is a battle cry against viruses, bacteria, and other pathogens that threaten your health.

The immune system is a complex network of cells, tissues, and organs working in concert to protect you. Picture white blood cells as the star soloists, patrolling the bloodstream and tissues, ready to respond at a moment's notice. Lymph nodes are the rehearsal spaces, where immune cells gather to prepare for their next performance. The thymus, spleen, and bone marrow are the training grounds, nurturing and educating the cells to recognize and combat invaders.

When a pathogen enters the body, it is like an unwelcome guest barging into a serene concert. The immune system's sensors, specialized cells like macrophages and dendritic cells detect the intruder and sound the alarm. This signal mobilizes the choir, with white blood cells rushing to the site of infection, much like singers taking their places on stage. This is exciting! Our human system is guarded and ought to remain that way. The purpose of this book is to enlighten the readers on the overall efforts they owe their bodies to keep the rhythm flowing. We are so privileged to have these machines working in us. Can we see the super work of God the Creator?

WHAT SILENCES THE CHOIR?
However, the immune system is not invincible. Several factors can dampen its powerful song, silencing the once-vibrant choir. Some of these factors are:

a-Chronic stress: This is like a constant dissonant note that disrupts the harmony. Prolonged exposure to stress hormones can weaken the immune response, making it harder for the body to fight off infections.

b-Poor nutrition: Another culprit that affects the functions of the immune system. Imagine trying to perform a complex piece without proper instruments or rehearsal time. A diet lacking in essential nutrients deprives the immune system of the tools it needs to function effectively. Vitamin deficiencies, particularly vitamins C and D, can impair the production and function of white blood cells.

c-Sleep: Sleep, or the lack thereof, also plays a critical role. Without adequate rest, the body struggles to repair and regenerate, leaving the immune system fatigued and less responsive. It is like expecting a choir to deliver a flawless performance after being awake all night, they simply can't give their best.

d-Autoimmune diseases: In these conditions, the immune system turns against itself, attacking healthy tissues as if they were foreign invaders. It is as though the choir becomes confused, misinterpreting the score and creating discord instead of harmony.

HOW TO BOOST YOUR IMMUNE RESPONSE

All is not lost. With the right strategies, you can strengthen your immune system and ensure the choir sings loudly and clearly. Here are steps to take:

a-A balanced diet: Start with a balanced diet rich in fruits, whole grains, vegetables, and lean proteins. These foods provide the vitamins, minerals, and antioxidants needed to fuel the immune response.

b-Exercise: Regular exercise is another key. It is like a rehearsal session that keeps the choir in peak condition. Physical activity enhances circulation, allowing immune cells to move freely throughout the body and do their job more effectively.

c-Adequate sleep: Prioritize sleep, aiming for 7-9 hours per night. Think of sleep as a restorative pause, giving your immune system the chance to regroup and prepare for the next performance. During sleep, the body produces cytokines, proteins that help fight infection and inflammation.

d-Reduce stress: Manage stress through mindfulness practices, meditation, or simply taking time each day to relax and unwind. Reducing stress is like tuning an instrument, ensuring each note is clear and precise.

e-Vaccination: Consider vaccinations as essential training sessions for your immune system. Vaccines expose the immune system to a harmless form of a pathogen, teaching it to recognize and respond quickly to future encounters.

By nurturing your immune system, you ensure that the body's defense choir remains strong and vibrant, ready to protect you from whatever threats come its way. Listen to your body's signals, support its needs, and let the harmonious song of health resonate within you.

A HARMONIOUS BODY

Congratulations to you dear reader for coming down to this junction.

We have probed into the operation of the delicate organs of our body working together in unity to upkeep our body balance. You have seen their functions, challenges, and proving ways they can be tuned back. Working today in harmony,

these organs serve us with full force but when they are interrupted, we cry out in pain. Each system, organ, and component of our body plays a vital role in maintaining overall health and functionality. Just as each instrument in an orchestra must be finely tuned and well-cared for to create beautiful music, our bodies require attention, care, and nurturing to perform at their best.

By understanding how our bodies work, what can hinder their functions, and how to maintain their health, we empower ourselves to live healthier, and more vibrant. Let the voice of your body guide you toward making informed decisions, adopting healthy habits, and embracing a lifestyle that supports complete wellness. Your body is speaking; listen to it, nurture it, and let it thrive.In the upcoming chapters,we will dive into the language and signs from our body's orchestra. What do they say when their activities are benefitting us? And what on earth do we hear from them immediately when they get interrupted? Let's find out!

CHAPTER TWELVE

THE BODY'S LANGUAGE

Signs and symptoms

Our bodies communicate with us through various signs and symptoms, signaling when something is amiss. Each sign or symptom corresponds to specific organs or systems, offering clues about underlying health issues. Understanding these messages can help us respond appropriately to maintain optimal health. Below are the noted signs and symptoms we receive from our body's great team:

1-PAIN

The Alarm bell

Pain is a complex and essential signal, serving as the body's alarm bell. It alerts us to potential harm or injury, prompting us to take action. Pain can be acute (short-term) or chronic (long-term), and it varies in intensity and location.

COMMON TYPES OF PAIN AND THEIR SOURCES:

a-Headache: This type is often linked to stress, dehydration, eye strain, or underlying conditions like migraines or sinus infections.

b-Chest pain: Can indicate heart issues, such as angina or heart attack, but can also be related to respiratory problems, acid reflux, or muscular strain.

c-Abdominal pain: This may signal digestive issues like indigestion, gastritis, or more severe conditions like appendicitis or gallstones.

d-Back pain: Often associated with musculoskeletal problems, poor posture, or kidney issues.

e-Joint Pain:Commonly related to arthritis, injuries, or autoimmune conditions.

There are others too, but we want to concentrate on these for the purpose of this book.

HOW DO WE RESPOND TO PAIN?

To manage and alleviate pain, consider these approaches:

a-Rest and Recovery: Allow time for healing and avoid activities that exacerbate pain.

b-Medication: Use pain relievers or prescribed medications as directed by a healthcare professional. Do not adapt to self prescription. You can worsen the pain by doing so.

c-Physical therapy: Engage in exercises and therapies to strengthen and support affected areas.

d-Lifestyle changes: Address underlying causes like poor posture, stress, or diet.

e-Medical Evaluation: Seek professional advice for persistent or severe pain to diagnose and treat underlying conditions.

2-FATIGUE
The Body's exhaustion

Fatigue is a common symptom that indicates physical or mental exhaustion. Unlike normal tiredness, fatigue persists even after rest and can significantly impact daily functioning.

CAUSES OF FATIGUE:

a-Sleep disorders: Conditions like insomnia, sleep apnea, or restless leg syndrome can disrupt restorative sleep.

b-Nutritional deficiencies: Lack of essential nutrients like iron, vitamin B12, or vitamin D can lead to fatigue.

c-Chronic illnesses: Diseases like diabetes, heart disease, and chronic fatigue syndrome often cause persistent tiredness.

d-Mental health issues: Depression, anxiety, and stress can drain energy levels and lead to fatigue.

e-Medications: Certain drugs, such as antihistamines, antidepressants, and blood pressure medications, can cause drowsiness.

HOW TO COMBAT FATIGUE

To address fatigue and restore energy, consider these strategies:

a-Improve sleep hygiene: Establish a regular sleep schedule, create a restful environment, and limit caffeine and screen time before bed.

b-Balanced diet: Eat a nutrient-rich diet, including iron, vitamins, and proteins, to support energy levels.

c-Regular exercise: Engage in physical activity to boost energy and improve overall health.

d-Stress management: Practice relaxation techniques like meditation, yoga, or deep breathing exercises.

e-Medical consultation: Seek professional advice to identify and treat underlying health issues causing fatigue.

3-FEVER
The heat of the battle

Fever is a rise in body temperature, typically indicating an immune response to infection. It is a natural defense mechanism, helping the body fight off pathogens by creating an inhospitable environment for bacteria and viruses.

COMMON CAUSES OF FEVER:

a-Infections: Bacterial, viral, or fungal infections are the most common causes of fever.

b-Inflammatory conditions: Autoimmune diseases like rheumatoid arthritis or inflammatory bowel disease can cause fever.

c-Heat exhaustion: Prolonged exposure to high temperatures or strenuous activity can lead to heat-related illnesses.

d-Medications and Vaccinations: Certain drugs and vaccines can trigger fever as a side effect.

HOW TO MANAGE FEVER:

To control fever and support the body's healing process, follow these guidelines:

a-Hydration: Drink plenty of fluids to prevent dehydration and help regulate body temperature.

b-Rest: Allow the body to recover by getting adequate rest and avoiding strenuous activities.

c-Cool Environment: Stay in a cool, comfortable environment and use lightweight clothing.

d-Medication: Use fever reducers as directed by your health provider. Seek professional help for persistent or high fever, especially in children, the elderly, or individuals with underlying health conditions.

4-SWELLING

Swelling, or edema, is the accumulation of fluid in tissues, causing them to become puffy and enlarged. It often indicates an underlying issue, such as injury, infection, or chronic disease.

COMMON CAUSES OF SWELLING:

a-Injury: Injuries such as sprains or fractures, can cause localized swelling.

b-Infections: Bacterial or viral infections can lead to swelling in affected areas.

c-Chronic conditions: Heart failure, kidney disease, and liver disease can cause widespread edema.

d-Allergic reactions: Allergies can trigger swelling, particularly in the face, lips, and airways.

e-Medications: Certain drugs, like corticosteroids and blood pressure medications, can cause fluid retention and swelling.

HOW TO REDUCE SWELLING

To manage and reduce swelling, consider these approaches:

a-Rest and Elevation: Elevate the affected area to reduce fluid accumulation and promote drainage.

b-Cold compress: Apply ice packs to the swollen area to reduce inflammation and pain. Use compression garments or bandages to support the affected area and reduce swelling.

a-Hydration: Drink plenty of water to help flush excess fluids from the body.

b-Medical advice: Consult a healthcare professional for persistent or severe swelling to identify and treat the underlying cause.

5-RASH
The Skin's signal

A rash is a change in the skin's appearance, often characterized by redness, itching, and irritation. It can result from various causes, ranging from mild irritants to serious medical conditions.

COMMON CAUSES OF RASHES

a-Allergies: Allergic reactions to foods, medications, or environmental factors can cause rashes.

b-Infections: Viral infections like chickenpox and measles, as well as bacterial infections like impetigo, can lead to rashes.

c-Skin conditions: Eczema, psoriasis, and contact dermatitis are common dermatological conditions that cause rashes.

d-Heat and Sweat: Heat rash occurs when sweat ducts become blocked, leading to irritation.

e-Medications: Certain medications can cause rashes as a side effect.

HOW TO TREAT RASHES

To treat rashes, follow these guidelines:

a-Avoid irritants: Identify and avoid allergens or irritants that trigger the rash.

b-Topical treatments: Use creams or ointments, to reduce itching and inflammation.

c-Cool compress: Apply cool, damp cloths to the affected area to soothe irritation.

d-Proper Hygiene: Keep the skin clean and dry to prevent further irritation and infection.

e-Medical Attention: Seek professional advice for severe, persistent, or spreading rashes to determine the underlying cause and appropriate treatment.

6-SHORTNESS OF BREATH
The body's call for air

Shortness of breath, or dyspnea, is a sensation of difficulty breathing. It can be a symptom of various health issues, ranging from respiratory conditions to cardiovascular problems.

COMMON CAUSES

a-Asthma: Chronic inflammation and narrowing of the airways can cause shortness of breath, especially during physical activity or exposure to allergens.

b-Chronic Obstructive Pulmonary Disease (COPD): Conditions like emphysema and chronic bronchitis can restrict airflow and lead to breathing difficulties.

c-Heart Conditions: Heart failure and other cardiovascular issues can cause fluid buildup in the lungs, leading to shortness of breath.

d-Infections: Respiratory infections like pneumonia and bronchitis can impair lung function and cause breathing problems.

e-Anxiety: Panic attacks and anxiety disorders can trigger a feeling of breathlessness.

ADDRESSING SHORTNESS OF BREATH

To alleviate shortness of breath, consider these strategies:

a-Controlled Breathing: Practice breathing exercises, such as diaphragmatic breathing, to improve lung function and reduce anxiety.

b-Medication: Use prescribed inhalers or medications to manage underlying respiratory conditions.

c-Avoid triggers: Identify and avoid allergens or irritants that worsen breathing difficulties.

d-Regular exercise: Engage in regular physical activity to strengthen respiratory muscles and improve overall lung capacity.

e-Medical evaluation: Seek professional advice for persistent or severe shortness of breath to diagnose and treat the underlying cause. Follow it up as early as possible to avoid chronic stage.

7- DIZZINESS

The body's balance alert

Dizziness is a sensation of lightheadedness, unsteadiness, or spinning. It can result from various causes, ranging from benign to serious medical conditions.

COMMON CAUSES OF DIZZINESS:

a-Dehydration: Inadequate fluid intake can lead to dizziness and lightheadedness.

b-Inner ear issues: Conditions like vertigo and labyrinthitis affect the inner ear, causing balance problems and dizziness.

c-Low blood pressure: Sudden drops in blood pressure, known as orthostatic hypotension, can cause dizziness.

d-Medications: Certain drugs, such as blood pressure medications and sedatives, can cause dizziness as a side effect.

e-Anemia: Low levels of red blood cells or hemoglobin can reduce oxygen delivery to the brain, leading to dizziness.

MANAGING DIZZINESS

To manage and reduce dizziness, consider these tips:

a-Hydration: Drink plenty of fluids to prevent dehydration, which can cause dizziness.

b-Move slowly: When standing up or changing positions, do so gradually to avoid sudden drops in blood pressure.

c-Avoid triggers: Identify and avoid factors that trigger dizziness, such as certain foods, medications, or activities.

d-Rest: Lie down in a dark, quiet room if you experience severe dizziness or vertigo, and avoid driving or operating machinery.

e-Balance exercises: Engage in exercises that improve balance and coordination, such as yoga or tai chi.

f-Medical consultation: Seek professional advice for persistent or severe dizziness to diagnose and treat the underlying cause.

8-NAUSEA
The Stomach's rebellion

Nausea is an uncomfortable sensation often accompanied by the urge to vomit. It can result from various causes, including digestive issues, infections, and motion sickness.

COMMON CAUSES OF NAUSEA

a-Gastrointestinal issues: Conditions like gastroenteritis, ulcers, and acid reflux can cause nausea.

b-Pregnancy: Morning sickness is a common symptom during the first trimester of pregnancy.

c-Medications: Certain drugs, such as chemotherapy agents and antibiotics, can cause nausea as a side effect.

d-Motion sickness: Travel by car, boat, or plane can trigger nausea in some individuals.

e-Infections: Viral or bacterial infections, particularly those affecting the digestive system, can cause nausea.

ALLEVIATING NAUSEA

To manage and alleviate nausea, consider these options:

a-Ginger: Consume ginger in various forms, such as tea, candy, or supplements, to help soothe nausea.

b-Small meals: Eat small, frequent meals rather than large ones to avoid overwhelming the digestive system.

c-Stay Hydrated: Sip on clear fluids like water, herbal tea, or electrolyte solutions to stay hydrated.

d-Rest and Relaxation: Rest in a comfortable position and practice deep breathing or relaxation techniques to reduce nausea.

e-Avoid triggers: Identify and avoid foods, smells, or activities that trigger nausea.

f-Medical advice: Consult a healthcare professional for persistent or severe nausea to identify and treat the underlying cause.

9-WEIGHT CHANGES

The Scale's message

Unexpected weight gain or loss can signal various health issues. Monitoring weight changes helps identify potential problems early.

COMMON CAUSES OF WEIGHT GAIN:

a-Overeating: Consuming more calories than the body needs can lead to weight gain.

b-Hypothyroidism: An underactive thyroid gland can slow metabolism and cause weight gain.

c-Medications: Certain drugs, such as corticosteroids and antidepressants, can cause weight gain as a side effect.

d-Sedentary lifestyle: Lack of physical activity contributes to weight gain and obesity.

e-Fluid retention: Conditions like heart failure, kidney disease, and liver disease can cause the body to retain fluids, leading to weight gain.

COMMON CAUSES OF WEIGHT LOSS:
a-Poor diet: Inadequate calorie intake or malnutrition can lead to weight loss.
b-Hyperthyroidism: An overactive thyroid gland increases metabolism, causing weight loss.
c-Chronic illness: Diseases like cancer, tuberculosis, and HIV/AIDS can cause significant weight loss.
d-Digestive disorders: Conditions like celiac disease, Crohn's disease, and ulcers can affect nutrient absorption, leading to weight loss.
e-Mental health issues: Depression, anxiety, and eating disorders can result in weight loss.

HOW TO MANAGE WEIGHT CHANGES

To address unexpected weight changes, consider these approaches:

a-Balanced diet: Consume a well-rounded diet rich in essential nutrients, including proteins, fats, and carbohydrates.

b-Regular exercise: Engage in regular physical activity to maintain a healthy weight and improve overall health.

c-Monitor weight: Keep track of weight changes and consult a healthcare professional if you notice significant fluctuations.

d-Medical evaluation: Seek professional advice for persistent or unexplained weight changes to diagnose and treat underlying health issues.

10-CHANGES IN APPETITE

The Hunger Signal

Changes in appetite, either increased or decreased, can indicate various health conditions or emotional states.

COMMON CAUSES OF INCREASED APPETITE:

a-Physical activity: Increased physical activity levels can boost appetite as the body demands more energy.

b-Medications: Certain drugs, such as steroids and some antidepressants, can increase appetite.

c-Hormonal changes: Hormonal fluctuations, such as those during puberty or pregnancy, can affect appetite.

d-Emotional factors: Stress, anxiety, and boredom can lead to emotional eating and increased appetite.

COMMON CAUSES OF DECREASED APPETITE:
a-Illness: Infections, chronic diseases, and certain cancers can reduce appetite.
b-Medications: Some drugs can decrease appetite. Always seek professional health care.
c-Mental health issues: Depression, anxiety, and eating disorders can suppress appetite.
d-Digestive disorders: Conditions like gastritis, ulcers, and irritable bowel syndrome can affect appetite.

MANAGING APPETITE CHANGES
To address changes in appetite, consider these strategies:
a-Balanced diet:Maintain a healthy diet to ensure adequate nutrient intake, even with appetite changes.
b-Regular meals: Stick to a regular eating schedule to help regulate appetite and ensure consistent nutrition.
c-Stress management: Practice techniques that helps in reducing stress such as mindfulness, meditation, and exercises to manage emotional eating.
d-Medical advice: Seek professional help for persistent or severe changes in appetite to identify and treat underlying causes.

LISTENING AND RESPONDING

Your body's feedback loop

Every great conductor knows how to listen to the orchestra and adjust the performance accordingly. Your body is constantly giving you signals, small cues that something might be off or needs attention. This is your body's feedback loop, and listening to it is crucial for maintaining health.

When you feel fatigued, stressed, or experience discomfort, it is your body's way of telling you to make an adjustment. Ignoring these signals is like continuing to play an out-of-tune instrument, which only leads to more significant problems down the road. By paying attention and responding, you can correct the course before it affects your entire performance.

The symphony of your body is never static, it is an evolving masterpiece. As you age, your body changes, and your health needs shift.

Continuous learning about how your body works and adapting your wellness practices accordingly ensures that you stay in tune with your body's needs.

This means being open to trying new exercises, incorporating different foods, and adjusting your routine as necessary. Just as an orchestra evolves with new compositions and techniques, so too must you adapt your health practices. By staying curious and committed, you allow your body's symphony to flourish, ensuring a lifetime of harmonious health.

Our bodies communicate with us through various signs and symptoms, each offering valuable insights into our health. By understanding and responding to these messages, we can take proactive steps to maintain our well-being. Remember, your body speaks to you every day. Listen carefully, respond thoughtfully, and embrace a lifestyle that supports complete wellness.

The journey to understanding and nurturing our bodies is ongoing. As we tune into the body's language, we learn to appreciate the intricate symphony of health that plays within us. By paying attention to the signs and symptoms, making informed decisions, and adopting healthy habits, we can create a harmonious balance that supports a vibrant, fulfilling life. Your body is your greatest ally, cherish it, care for it, and let it guide you toward a healthier future.

CHAPTER THIRTEEN

NUTRITION, HYDRATION AND EXERCISE

Imagine your body's orchestra running low on energy, its instruments out of tune, and the melody faltering. Food is more than fuel; it is the sheet music that guides the performance. Every bite you take is a note added to the grand score. Carbohydrates, fats, and proteins are the main players, but without the harmony provided by vitamins and minerals, the music loses its clarity. The heart's drumbeat weakens, the digestive bass section rumbles out of sync, and your muscles' strings go limp.

A balanced diet feeds the orchestra with what it needs to play at its best. Whole foods like fruits, vegetables, lean meats, and grains act as the conductor's baton, keeping each player in line. They provide the nutrients that empower your heart to keep drumming, your lungs to keep fluting, and your immune system to raise its chorus against invaders.

FOODS THAT HARM AND FOODS THAT HEAL

The orchestra can be sabotaged by junk food, processed sugars, trans fats, and artificial additives that bring nothing but discord. They clog your arteries, weaken the conductor (your nervous system), and send the immune choir into a sluggish, offbeat performance.

But then, healing foods like berries, leafy greens, and healthy fats enter the stage. These are the heroes that repair damage, re-energize tired sections, and restore balance. When you eat right, your body hums with perfect pitch. The strings of your muscles tighten, the drummer (your heart) beats strong, and the flutes (your lungs) fill with the breath of life. Give your body what it yearns for and it can keep you miles away from frequent visits to the clinic and overuse of medications.

HYDRATION
The life-giving water

Have you seen an orchestra playing in the desert, parched, dry, and struggling? Water is not just a backdrop; it is the river on which your body's music flows. Without it, the instruments start to warp. Your skin dries out, the heart slows, and your brain, the master conductor, becomes foggy and disoriented.

Hydration is the key to fluidity in every bodily function. Water lubricates the strings of your muscles, moistens the flutes of your lungs, and keeps the percussion of your skeletal system flexible. Every cell relies on water to vibrate with life, ensuring that each note played is crisp and clear.

SIGNS OF DEHYDRATION AND HOW TO PREVENT IT

Dehydration does not strike like a loud cymbal crash; it is a gradual, quiet dissonance. It starts with dry lips, headaches, or dizziness-the whisper of instruments out of tune. Your digestive bass becomes sluggish, your heart's drum loses rhythm, and the skin's protective barrier weakens, making you vulnerable to outside invaders.

Preventing dehydration is simple: drink water before your body's music falters. Keep a bottle of water nearby throughout the day, and tune into your body's cues. If you feel tired, lightheaded, or notice dark urine, your body is sending you signals that it is drying out. Keep your orchestra hydrated, and the performance stays smooth.

EXERCISES
Keeping the instruments in shape
Exercise is the rehearsal that keeps every part of the orchestra in top form. It is the daily practice that ensures the strings of your muscles do not slacken, the heart's beat remains strong, and the lungs can produce a steady melody. Without regular activity, the music fades into lethargy, each section becoming stiff and out of sync.

Regular exercise brings every instrument to life. Aerobic exercises pump oxygen through your body like wind through flutes, while strength training reinforces the strings of your muscles. Flexibility exercises like yoga and stretching keep your joints, the percussion section, lumber and ready to strike at a moment's notice. Each movement is a tune-up, ensuring your body is always ready for its next grand performance.

TYPES OF EXERCISES FOR DIFFERENT BODY SYSTEMS

Each section of your orchestra requires a unique kind of exercise. Cardio activities like walking or swimming feed oxygen to your heart and lungs, keeping the rhythm fast and powerful. Strength training focuses on tightening the strings of your muscles, while stretching exercises ensure your joints can withstand any pressure. Balance exercises help the nervous system, the conductor, to keep directing without hesitation or faltering.

By combining different exercises, you are rehearsing the full symphony. This prepares your body for the physical and mental demands of life, allowing each system to play its part in perfect harmony. I hope that you are taking note of all these. The "Voice Of Your Body" is masterfully designed to equip you to possess back all you have you have lost in your health journey. Remember that it is never too late to build back again.

REST
The recharging breaks

Exercise and sleep are like twin sisters. You cannot take one and leave the other. Even the greatest orchestra needs breaks between performances. Rest is not a luxury, it is a necessity. Without it, the instruments break, the musicians tire, and the entire composition falls apart. Sleep is when the body's true restoration happens. Muscles repair themselves, the immune system strengthens its defenses, and the brain processes the day's events, preparing for the next performance.

When you skip rest, your body begins to falter. The heart's steady beat becomes erratic, the muscles weaken, and your nervous system, the conductor, loses focus.

Rest is the rehearsal for a stronger tomorrow, allowing every system to recharge and prepare for another day of harmonious performance.

HOW LACK OF REST AFFECTS THE BODY

A lack of rest is like trying to play an instrument with broken strings or a torn drum. Sleep deprivation dulls the entire orchestra. Your immune system's choir becomes too tired to fight, your heart's drum slows its beat, and your nervous system loses its sharpness. The melody of your body fades, leaving you vulnerable to sickness, fatigue, and stress.

By allowing your body to rest through deep sleep, relaxation techniques, and even meditation, you give it the chance to repair, rebuild, and recharge. Just as an orchestra needs downtime to fine-tune its instruments, your body requires rest to maintain its peak performance.

CHAPTER FOURTEEN

MENTAL HEALTH

The Silent Maestro

Your mental health is the invisible maestro guiding the performance of your body. Stress, anxiety, and negative emotions are like background noise that throws the entire orchestra out of sync. The heart begins to race, the muscles tighten in anxiety, and the immune system falters under the pressure.

On the other hand, a calm and clear mind sharpens the conductor's baton. It allows the body to flow in perfect rhythm, directing the heart, lungs, and muscles in harmony. A positive mental state is like the melody that gives life to the entire performance.

There are simple yet powerful techniques to keep your mental health in check.

a-Mindfulness, meditation, and breathing exercises clear the static, allowing your body to function as one united orchestra. These practices slow the heart rate, relax the muscles, and sharpen the brain. It is like giving your conductor a fresh baton, ready to lead with precision.

By caring for your mental health, you ensure that the performance does not just survive, it thrives, with each system playing its part in perfect tune.

MIND-BODY CONNECTION

Practices that promote harmony

The mind and body are not separate players, they are a duet that must work together. Your thoughts and emotions influence how your body performs, and your physical health directly impacts your mental well-being. This is the core of the mind-body connection, where every emotion, stressor, or mental shift sends ripples through your body's systems.

Practices like yoga, Tai Chi, and meditation are ways to bring this duet into harmony. These exercises allow your mind to calm, which in turn relaxes your muscles, slows your heart, and clears your lungs. When the mind is centered, the body follows, and the entire orchestra plays in sync.

BENEFITS OF MINDFULNESS AND MEDITATION

Mindfulness and meditation are like tuning your mind to the perfect pitch. These practices help you focus on the present moment, clearing away the distractions and stresses that throw your body's performance off. Just like a conductor guiding each musician, your mind becomes the guide, keeping every system in check. When you meditate, your body responds, your heart rate lowers, your breathing deepens, and your muscles relax. Regular mindfulness practices improve not just your mental state but your physical health as well. They are the quiet moments of reflection that allow your body to return to its natural rhythm, setting the stage for peak performance

CREATING A HEALTHY LIFESTYLE ROUTINE

Daily habits for a balanced life

Your body's orchestra does not just perform once, it plays every single day. The key to a balanced life is creating a routine where each system, from the heart to the brain, knows when and how to perform. The daily habits you form are like the conductor's steady hand, ensuring that your body's symphony flows smoothly.

From what you eat in the morning to how you wind down at night, every choice you make is a note in the composition. Eating nutritious meals, staying active, hydrating, and getting restful sleep, all these are vital pieces of the puzzle. When combined, they create harmony, allowing your heart to beat strong, your lungs to breathe easily, and your mind to stay sharp.

The best performances are built on practice and progression. Setting unrealistic goals, like trying to overhaul your entire lifestyle in one day, is like demanding a flawless concert without a single rehearsal. Start small and build gradually.

For example, begin by adding 10 minutes of stretching to your mornings, or substitute one unhealthy snack for a nutritious one. Every small change brings your body closer to playing in perfect harmony. Over time, these small adjustments become second nature, turning your routine into a seamless and sustainable symphony of health.

CONCLUSION

Embracing the symphony of your body

As we reach the final movement of this symphony, it is time to reflect on the remarkable masterpiece that is, your body. Every breath, heartbeat, and muscle contraction plays a role in this delicate, harmonious composition that has been with you from the very beginning. Each system, each function, and each signal works together in perfect rhythm to keep you alive, healthy, and thriving. This book has been a journey through the fundamental workings of your body's orchestra, but now it is time to bring everything together and embrace the symphony of your health in its entirety.

CELEBRATING YOUR BODY'S INNATE WISDOM

Your body is far more than just a collection of systems working in isolation, it is a living, breathing symphony that performs tirelessly, day in and day out, to keep you functioning at your best. The heart drums a steady beat, the lungs sing a melody of life-giving air, the muscles stretch and contract like strings on an instrument, and the brain conducts the entire performance with effortless precision.

This process is not something we always appreciate. We often forget the extraordinary complexity behind the seemingly simple acts of walking, breathing, or thinking. But your body is always there, adapting and adjusting to meet your needs, whether you are aware of it or not. It is time to celebrate this innate wisdom that is built into you, a wisdom that knows exactly how to heal wounds, fight infections, digest food, and power your every move. We thank God for this!

When you take a moment to really listen, you can hear your body speaking in the language of sensations, subtle whispers of hunger, thirst, fatigue, or energy. Your body knows what it needs, and it is always guiding you toward balance. All you have to do is listen.

LISTENING TO THE VOICE OF YOUR BODY

Learning to listen to your body is like learning to tune an instrument. It requires attention, practice, and patience. But the more you attune yourself to its signals, the better you become at recognizing when something is out of sync. You might start noticing how your energy dips when you are dehydrated or how stress tightens your muscles and speeds up your heart rate. Perhaps you begin to understand the ways in which your emotions influence your digestion or how a lack of sleep makes you more vulnerable to illness.

Your body is constantly communicating with you, sending messages in the form of sensations, discomfort, pain, or pleasure. These signals are your body's way of letting you know what it needs, and by tuning in to these signals, you can respond in a way that supports your health. It can be adjusting your diet, increasing your physical activity, or simply taking a moment to rest. Listening to your body allows you to take proactive steps toward maintaining balance and harmony.

THE IMPORTANCE OF BALANCE AND HARMONY

Just like an orchestra needs balance between its instruments to produce beautiful music, your body needs balance between its systems to function optimally. Too much of one thing, be it stress, unhealthy foods, or lack of sleep, can disrupt the delicate harmony and throw your body out of tune. This is why it is so important to cultivate balance in all areas of your life, from nutrition and exercise to mental health and self-care.

Your journey to health does not have to be about perfection; it is about balance. Some days, your symphony may not sound flawless, and that's okay. What is important is the overall harmony you cultivate over time, adjusting when necessary, just like an orchestra tunes its instruments before every performance. Life will always bring challenges, but your body has an incredible ability to adapt and bounce back, especially when you nurture it with care and respect.

A LIFELONG PROCESS

This book has guided you through the various systems that make up the body's symphony, but the journey does not end here. The real symphony is ongoing, and your role as the conductor is lifelong. You have learned about the heart's rhythm, the lungs' melody, the muscles' strength, and the nervous system's direction. Now it is time to apply that knowledge in your daily life.

Developing a healthy relationship with your body is a continuous process. Just as a musician practices to stay in tune, you must continuously check in with your body and make adjustments to keep everything running smoothly. This means staying mindful of your nutrition, exercise, mental health, and rest. It also means being compassionate with yourself, having the

understanding that some days your body might not perform perfectly, but that is part of the journey.

Taking time to rest, nourish yourself, move your body, and engage in activities that bring you joy are all essential parts of keeping the symphony alive. Self-care is the tuning process that keeps your instruments ready for the long haul.

REFLECTIONS

Reflection also plays a crucial role in maintaining this harmony. By regularly reflecting on how your body feels, what it needs, and how you can support it, helps deepen your understanding of yourself. Are you feeling sluggish because of poor sleep? Is your digestive system off because of stress? Is your heart racing because you have been overworking yourself? Reflection helps you adjust your routine to better serve your body's needs.

The symphony of your body does not have an ending, it is a continuous, ever-evolving masterpiece. It changes as you age, adapts to new challenges, and adjusts to the rhythms of life. While the tempo may slow down with time and certain notes may change, the music never stops. The beauty of this symphony is in its resilience and its ability to keep playing, no matter what life throws your way.

By embracing the beat of your body, you are not just passively experiencing life, you are actively participating in your health. You are the conductor, and every decision you make, every habit you cultivate, contributes to the quality of the performance. It is not about striving for perfection but about creating a life where your body can thrive in balance and harmony.

In conclusion, your body is an extraordinary composition, a living, breathing symphony that deserves to be celebrated. By listening, responding, and caring for it, you allow it to perform at its best. You have the power to shape your health, to guide your body's orchestra toward a life filled with vitality, energy, and well-being. So, embrace the voice of your body, honor its wisdom, and let the music of your life play on with grace and strength.

ABOUT THE AUTHOR

Damaris Roberts is a passionate advocate for health and fitness, specializing in crafting accessible and transformative exercise programs for individuals. With a career spanning over the years in the wellness industry, Damaris has dedicated her life to empowering seniors and others to embrace a more active and fulfilling lifestyle.

Driven by a deep understanding of the unique challenges faced by human folks, especially older adults, her approach combines expert knowledge with compassion and practical advice.

Damaris' writing is characterized by its clear, engaging style, making complex health concepts easy to understand and apply. She is committed to helping seniors achieve their fitness goals, improve their quality of life, and inspire them to live their best years with vitality and confidence.

Connect with Damaris Roberts to stay updated on the latest books, tips, and resources for a healthier, happier you.

YOUR FEEDBACK

Dear readers, your feedback is invaluable. If you have found this book helpful or have suggestions for improvement, please share your thoughts. Your experiences can inspire and assist others on their life's journey.

Your dedication to your health is commendable, and I wish you all the best as you continue to explore and benefit from "The Voice Of Your Body".

Kindly drop your positive reviews for this book as it motivates me in my publishing journey. Thank you!

OTHER BOOKS BY DAMARIS ROBERTS

1- Yoga Exercises For Seniors Over 60
2- Somatic Exercises For Seniors Over 60
3- Core Exercises And Nutrition For Seniors Over 60
4- Stress - Relief Exercises For Seniors Over 60
5- Intermittent Fasting For Seniors Over 60
6- Your Transformative Journey To A Healthier And A Happier Life

www.ingramcontent.com/pod-product-compliance
Lightning Source LLC
Chambersburg PA
CBHW071101240526
45471CB00016B/2290